SMOOTHIE FOR COLITIS

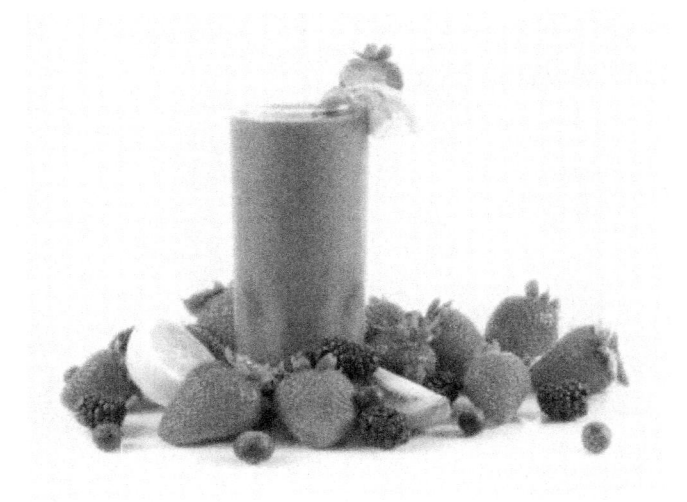

DR. JESSICA SMITH

Copyright © 2022 by Dr. Jessica Smith

All rights reserved.

No part of this publication may be reproduced, distributed, or transmitted in any form or by any means, including photocopying, recording, or other electronic or mechanical methods, without the prior written permission of the publisher, except in the case of brief quotations embodied in critical reviews and certain other non-commercial uses permitted by copyright law.

TABLE OF CONTENT

INTRODUCTION 7

CHAPTER ONE 9

   What are smoothies? 9

   Types of smoothies 11

   Benefits of consuming healthy Smoothies 14

   Disadvantages of consuming smoothies 16

CHAPTER TWO 19

   What is colitis? 19

   Types of colitis 19

   General symptoms of colitis 22

   Health benefits of drinking smoothie for colitis 24

CHAPTER THREE 26

   Smoothie recipes for colitis disease 26

   1. Blueberry Banana Smoothie: 26

   2. Mango Pineapple Smoothie: 27

   3. Peanut Butter Banana Smoothie: 27

   4. Carrot Orange Smoothie: 28

   5. Avocado Mango Smoothie: 29

   6. Green Apple Smoothie: 30

   7. Spinach Strawberry Smoothie: 30

   8. Kiwi Coconut Smoothie: 31

   9. Pineapple Banana Smoothie: 32

10. Beet Apple Smoothie: 32

11. Kale Orange Smoothie: 33

12. Papaya Coconut Smoothie: 34

13. Peach Almond Smoothie: 35

14. Carrot Orange Ginger Smoothie: 35

15. Apple Cinnamon Smoothie: 36

16. Banana Oat Smoothie: 37

17. Strawberry Coconut Smoothie: 38

18. Watermelon Mint Smoothie: 38

19. Kale Banana Smoothie: 39

20. Avocado Pineapple Smoothie: 40

21. Blueberry Banana Colitis Smoothie: 41

22. Pineapple Mango Colitis Smoothie: 41

23. Spinach Kale Colitis Smoothie: 42

24. Green Apple Colitis Smoothie: 43

25. Strawberry Banana Colitis Smoothie: 43

26. Avocado Pear Colitis Smoothie: 44

27. Coconut Mango Colitis Smoothie: 44

28. Peach Blueberry Colitis Smoothie: 45

29. Apple Cinnamon Colitis Smoothie: 46

30. Lemon Ginger Colitis Smoothie: 46

31. Orange Carrot Colitis Smoothie: 47

32. Kale Banana Colitis Smoothie: 47

33. Cucumber Melon Colitis Smoothie: 48

34. Pineapple Coconut Colitis Smoothie: 49

35. Acai Berry Colitis Smoothie: 49

36. Mango Coconut Colitis Smoothie: 50

37. Banana Almond Butter Colitis Smoothie: 50

38. Carrot Orange Colitis Smoothie: 51

39. Peach Coconut Colitis Smoothie: 51

40. Strawberry Coconut Colitis Smoothie: 52

41. Green Colitis Smoothie: 52

42. Mango Turmeric Smoothie: 53

43. Blueberry Ginger Smoothie: 54

44. Coconut Berry Smoothie: 54

45. Avocado Spinach Smoothie: 55

46. Broccoli Beet Smoothie: 56

47. Carrot Apple Smoothie: 56

48. Kale Pineapple Smoothie: 57

49. Banana Oat Smoothie: 58

50. Sweet Potato Cucumber Smoothie: 58

51. Carrot Orange Smoothie: 59

52. Kale Coconut Smoothie: 60

53. Spinach Mango Smoothie: 60

54. Beet Ginger Smoothie: 61

55. Apple Banana Smoothie: 62

56. Cucumber Pineapple Smoothie: 62

57. Avocado Turmeric Smoothie: 63

58. Strawberry Hemp Smoothie: 64

59. Broccoli Coconut Smoothie: 64

60. Banana Chia Smoothie: 65

61. Tropical Colitis Smoothie - 66

62. Blueberry-Mango Colitis Smoothie - 66

63. Green Colitis Smoothie - 67

64. Coconut Colitis Smoothie - 68

65. Strawberry Colitis Smoothie - 68

66. Citrus Colitis Smoothie - 69

67. Pineapple Colitis Smoothie - 69

68. Avocado Colitis Smoothie - 70

69. Acai Colitis Smoothie - 71

70. Mango Colitis Smoothie - 71

71. Papaya Colitis Smoothie - 72

72. Peach Colitis Smoothie - 72

73. Watermelon Colitis Smoothie - 73

74. Raspberry Colitis Smoothie - 74

75. Carrot Colitis Smoothie - 74

76. Kale Colitis Smoothie - 75

77. Cucumber Colitis Smoothie - 75

78. Beet Colitis Smoothie - 76

79. Grape Colitis Smoothie - 77

80. Banana-Spinach Colitis Smoothie - 77

Conclusion 79

INTRODUCTION

Rihanna was once suffering from ulcerative colitis, a serious and debilitating chronic inflammatory bowel disease (IBD), but she successfully reversed the disease with a special smoothie.

For over a year, Rihanna followed a strict diet of smoothies, made up of fruits and vegetables, which she drank up to five times a day. She started with a smoothie that contained ingredients like kale, spinach, pineapple, ginger, and cucumber, as well as a probiotic powder and apple cider vinegar.

Rihanna then added other ingredients such as chia seeds, flaxseeds, lemon juice, and almond milk to her smoothie, to increase the nutritional value of the drink. She also incorporated natural supplements including turmeric, probiotics, and aloe vera, as well as herbs like chamomile and lavender, to enhance the healing potential of the smoothie.

In addition to the smoothie, Rihanna also followed a strict diet that consisted of only plant-based foods and eliminated all processed sugars, starches, and fats. She also cut out all dairy, gluten, and alcohol from her diet and eliminated any food that was processed or contained artificial ingredients.

Rihanna also incorporated exercise into her daily routine to help manage her symptoms and to help her body heal. She would do simple exercises such as walking, stretching, and yoga, and she also incorporated a light weight lifting routine.

Finally, Rihanna incorporated relaxation techniques such as deep breathing, meditation, and mindfulness into her daily routine. She also made sure to get enough sleep and rest, and she avoided stressful situations as much as possible.

Within a few months of following her program, Rihanna's ulcerative colitis was in remission and the symptoms of the disease had completely disappeared. Her story serves as an inspiring reminder that with the right diet and lifestyle changes, it is possible to reverse even the most severe chronic illnesses.

CHAPTER ONE

What are smoothies?

A smoothie is a thick, cold beverage made from pureed raw fruits or vegetables, often combined with juices, dairy products, nuts, seeds, and other ingredients. It is usually served in a glass or bowl and is a popular snack or breakfast option.

Smoothies are typically made with a base of fruit or vegetable puree, ice, and a liquid such as juice, milk, yogurt, or water. Additional ingredients can include honey, agave syrup, nut butter, protein powder, spices, and superfoods. Smoothies can be customized to suit individual tastes and dietary preferences.

Smoothies are a great way to get a nutritious and delicious snack or meal on the go. They are made with nutrient-rich fruits and vegetables and can be easily customized to suit individual dietary preferences.

Smoothies are a great way to get the recommended daily servings of fruits and vegetables, as well as protein, healthy fats, and other essential nutrients. They can also provide energy and help to keep cravings at bay.

Smoothies are easy to make and can be adapted to suit any dietary preferences or food allergies. They are also a great way to use up extra fruits and vegetables that are on the verge of going bad.

Smoothies can be made with fresh or frozen fruits and vegetables, so it is easy to keep a variety of ingredients on hand for quick and easy smoothies.

Smoothies are also a great way to sneak in extra servings of fruits and vegetables for picky eaters. They can be made with a variety of flavors and combinations, so it is easy to find something that appeals to everyone.

Smoothies are also a great way to get all of the essential vitamins and minerals that our bodies need. Smoothies can be a nutritious and convenient snack or meal and are a great way to get the recommended servings of fruits and vegetables.

They can be easily customized to suit individual dietary preferences and can be a great way to use up extra fruits and vegetables that are on the verge of going bad.

Smoothies are also a great way to sneak in extra servings of fruits and vegetables for picky eaters and can provide energy and help to keep cravings at bay.

In conclusion, smoothies are a great way to get a nutritious and delicious snack or meal on the go. They are made with nutrient-rich fruits and vegetables and can be easily customized to suit individual dietary preferences.

They are also an excellent way to get all of the essential vitamins and minerals our bodies need.

Types of smoothies

A smoothie is a blended, sometimes sweetened, beverage made from fresh fruit and/or vegetables, typically using a blender.

Smoothies can also include other ingredients such as water, crushed ice, frozen fruit, honey, dairy products, nuts, seeds, tea, chocolate, natural sweeteners, or nutritional supplements such as soy protein powder.

Smoothies are a great way to get a nutritious, balanced meal with minimal effort. They can be made with a variety of ingredients and customized to meet your individual needs and tastes. Here are some of the different types of smoothies you can make.

1. Green Smoothie – A blend of leafy green vegetables such as spinach, kale, or collard greens with other ingredients such as fruits, nuts, nut butter, and yogurt. This type of smoothie is high in vitamins, minerals, fiber, and antioxidants.

2. Protein Smoothie – This type of smoothie is typically higher in protein than other types of smoothies. It can contain ingredients such as whey protein powder, Greek yogurt, nut butter, and fruits and vegetables.

3. Detox Smoothie – A combination of ingredients that are designed to help your body detoxify and cleanse itself of toxins. Ingredients can include fruits, vegetables, nuts, seeds, and herbs.

4. Fruit Smoothie – A combination of fruits, juice, ice, and yogurt or milk. This type of smoothie can be high in sugar and calories, so it's important to watch portion sizes.

5. Nutrient-Packed Smoothie – This type of smoothie typically contains a variety of fruits, vegetables, nuts, seeds, and healthy fats.

These ingredients are packed with vitamins, minerals, and healthy fats that can help to boost your energy levels and provide nutrition.

6. Breakfast Smoothie – A combination of ingredients that can provide a quick and nutritious breakfast. Ingredients can include fruits, vegetables, yogurt, and protein powder.

7. Immune-Boosting Smoothie – This type of smoothie is designed to help support the immune system and can include ingredients such as ginger, turmeric, citrus fruits, and spinach.

8. Vegetable Smoothie – A combination of vegetables, fruits, and other ingredients that can provide a nutritious and filling meal or snack. Ingredients can include leafy greens, carrots, celery, and other vegetables.

9. Superfood Smoothie – A combination of nutrient-dense superfoods such as chia seeds, flaxseed, goji berries, and hemp seeds. This type of smoothie can be high in vitamins, minerals, and antioxidants.

10. Protein-Packed Smoothie – This type of smoothie is typically higher in protein than other types of smoothies.

It can contain ingredients such as whey protein powder, Greek yogurt, nut butter, and fruits and vegetables.

Benefits of consuming healthy Smoothies

Smoothies are a great way to get a wide variety of nutrients and vitamins into your daily diet. The combination of fruits, vegetables, dairy, and other ingredients makes for a delicious and nutritious snack or meal replacement. Here are some of the benefits of drinking healthy smoothies:

1. Improved Digestion: Smoothies are a great way to get essential fiber and other nutrients into your system. Fiber helps your body process food and can help to reduce bloating, constipation, and other digestive issues.

Adding fresh fruits, vegetables, and other ingredients to your smoothies helps to ensure that you get the vitamins, minerals, and fiber your body needs to stay healthy.

2. Boosted Immune System: Many smoothie ingredients are high in antioxidants, which are essential for a strong immune system. Fruits and vegetables like strawberries, blueberries, spinach, kale, and other greens are packed with vitamins and minerals that can help to boost your immunity. Adding yogurt or kefir to your smoothie can also provide beneficial probiotics, which are important for a healthy gut and overall immune system.

3. Increased Energy: Smoothies can provide a great energy boost throughout the day. Fruits and vegetables contain natural sugars that are slowly released into your system, giving you an extended energy boost that won't lead to any crashes.

Adding nuts and seeds to your smoothie can also provide a good source of healthy fats that can provide energy for hours.

4. Weight Loss: Smoothies are a great way to get a lot of nutrients into your system without consuming excess calories. Since smoothies are typically made from fresh fruits and vegetables, they are low in calories and fat.

Adding protein powder or nuts to your smoothie can also help to keep you full longer, making it easier to maintain a healthy weight.

Drinking healthy smoothies can be a great way to get a variety of essential nutrients into your system and can provide many health benefits. The combination of ingredients can provide you with an energy boost, improved digestion, a stronger immune system, and even help with weight loss.

Try to include a variety of fruits, vegetables, dairy, and other ingredients in your smoothies to get the most out of them. Experiment with different combinations to find out what works best for you and your body.

With the right ingredients, smoothies can be a delicious and nutritious addition to your diet.

Disadvantages of consuming smoothies

Smoothies are a popular choice for those looking for a quick and easy way to get their daily nutrients. While they can be a great way to get some healthy fruits and vegetables into your diet, there are a few potential disadvantages to consuming smoothies.

First, many smoothies contain added sugar. This can quickly add up, resulting in a high-calorie drink with no real nutritional benefit.

Additionally, many smoothies contain a lot of liquid, so the actual amount of nutrients in each serving can be quite low. If the smoothie is made with a lot of fruit juice, it can also contain a lot of empty calories.

Second, if you're making your own smoothies at home, it can be difficult to know exactly what nutrients you're getting.

There are also certain ingredients that can have a negative effect on your health if consumed in large amounts. For example, some smoothies contain a lot of added sugar, which can be hard on your teeth.

Additionally, some smoothies contain high amounts of caffeine, which can cause insomnia, anxiety, and other side effects.

Finally, consuming too many smoothies can lead to digestive issues. The high-fiber content of the fruits and vegetables in the smoothie can be difficult for some people to digest, leading to bloating and other digestive issues. Additionally, if the smoothie contains dairy, this can be hard for people with lactose intolerance to digest.

In conclusion, smoothies can be a great way to get some healthy nutrients into your diet. However, there are some potential disadvantages to consider, such as added sugar, low nutrient content, and digestive issues.

It's important to be mindful of the ingredients in your smoothie and to not overconsume them.

By being mindful of the potential disadvantages of consuming smoothies, you can ensure that you're getting the most out of your drink without compromising your health.

CHAPTER TWO

What is colitis?

Colitis is an inflammation of the inner lining of the colon, which is the large intestine. Depending on the cause, colitis may be acute (short-term) or chronic (long-term).

Symptoms of colitis can include abdominal pain and cramping, diarrhea (sometimes bloody), rectal pain, fatigue, weight loss, and fever. The most common causes of colitis vary, depending on the type.

Common causes of colitis include infection, irritable bowel syndrome (IBS), and inflammatory bowel disease (IBD). Treatment for colitis usually involves medications, diet modification, and lifestyle changes.

Types of colitis

1. Ulcerative Colitis: This type of colitis is characterized by ulcers that form in the inner lining of the colon. Symptoms may include bloody diarrhea, abdominal pain and cramping, fever, weight loss, and fatigue.

Treatment typically includes medications such as corticosteroids and immunomodulators, as well as lifestyle changes such as avoiding certain trigger foods and stress management.

2. Crohn's Disease: This is an inflammatory bowel disease that can affect any part of the gastrointestinal tract, but is most commonly found in the small intestine.

Symptoms include abdominal pain and cramping, bloody diarrhea, fatigue, and weight loss. Treatment typically includes medications such as corticosteroids, immunomodulators, and biologic therapies, along with lifestyle changes.

3. Infectious Colitis: This type of colitis is caused by bacterial or viral infections such as E. coli or Salmonella. Symptoms may include abdominal pain and cramping, bloody diarrhea, fever, and dehydration.

Treatment typically includes antibiotics and other medications, as well as lifestyle changes such as avoiding certain trigger foods.

4. Ischemic Colitis: This type of colitis occurs when there is decreased blood flow to the colon.

Symptoms may include abdominal pain and cramping, bloody diarrhea, and fever. Treatment typically includes medications such as anticoagulants and antiplatelet agents, as well as lifestyle changes such as increasing dietary fiber and avoiding certain trigger foods.

5. Collagenous Colitis: This type of colitis is characterized by thickening of the inner lining of the colon. Symptoms may include abdominal pain and cramping, bloody diarrhea, fever, and weight loss.

Treatment typically includes medications such as corticosteroids and immunomodulators, as well as lifestyle changes such as avoiding certain trigger foods and stress management.

6. Lymphocytic Colitis: This type of colitis is characterized by an increase in the number of lymphocytes in the colon. Symptoms may include abdominal pain and cramping, bloody diarrhea, and fatigue.

Treatment typically includes medications such as corticosteroids and immunomodulators, as well as lifestyle changes such as avoiding certain trigger foods and stress management.

7. Microscopic Colitis: This type of colitis is characterized by inflammation of the colon that cannot be seen with the naked eye. Symptoms may include abdominal pain and cramping, bloody diarrhea, and fatigue.

Treatment typically includes medications such as corticosteroids, immunomodulators, and biologics, as well as lifestyle changes such as avoiding certain trigger foods and stress management.

No matter what type of colitis you have, it is important to talk to your doctor about your symptoms and treatment options.

General symptoms of colitis

Colitis is a type of inflammatory bowel disease (IBD) that causes inflammation in the large intestine (colon). Symptoms of colitis can include cramping, abdominal pain, and bloody diarrhea.

Other symptoms may include urgency for bowel movements, fever, fatigue, loss of appetite, and weight loss. In some cases, people may experience abdominal bloating, rectal bleeding, and anemia.

The most common symptom of colitis is diarrhea, which can range from loose and watery to bloody stools. Cramping and abdominal pain are also common symptoms, and can range from mild to severe.

Other symptoms can include constipation, bloating, and fatigue. Some people may experience anemia, which can cause fatigue and paleness.

In some cases, people with colitis may experience other symptoms, such as joint pain, skin rashes, and eye inflammation. It is important to note that these symptoms are not always present in people with colitis.

People with colitis may also be more likely to develop infections and other complications, such as dehydration and malnutrition.

Colitis is typically treated with medications and lifestyle changes. Medications may include anti-inflammatory drugs, antibiotics, and immune system suppressants.

Diet and lifestyle changes can also help reduce symptoms and improve quality of life. These may include eating a well-balanced diet, getting regular exercise, and reducing stress. Surgery may also be an option for some people with colitis.

If you are experiencing any of the symptoms of colitis, it is important to seek medical attention as soon as possible. Early diagnosis and treatment can help reduce the severity of symptoms and reduce the risk of complications.

Health benefits of drinking smoothie for colitis

Colitis is a term that is commonly used to describe a group of gastrointestinal diseases, which can cause inflammation of the colon and rectum. While there is no one-size-fits-all treatment for colitis, drinking smoothies is one way to help manage the symptoms.

Smoothies are a great way to get the nutrients your body needs to stay healthy, while also helping to reduce inflammation.

Smoothies are made by blending fruits and vegetables, healthy fats, and other ingredients. This makes them an ideal way to get the vitamins, minerals, and other nutrients that are necessary for overall health. Smoothies are also an excellent source of dietary fiber, which can help to reduce inflammation in the digestive tract and ease some of the symptoms of colitis.

Smoothies can also help to reduce the symptoms of colitis by providing the body with probiotics. Probiotics are healthy bacteria that can help to restore balance in the digestive tract and improve the absorption of nutrients. This can help to reduce the inflammation that is associated with colitis.

Smoothies can also provide the body with essential amino acids that can help to reduce inflammation and improve gut health. Amino acids are the building blocks of proteins and are important for a healthy digestive system.

In addition, smoothies are a great way to get a boost of energy. This can help to reduce fatigue, which is a common symptom of colitis. Smoothies are also a great way to stay hydrated, which can help to reduce the amount of inflammation in the digestive tract.

Finally, smoothies can be a great way to get your daily intake of vitamins and minerals. This can help to support overall health and reduce the risk of developing colitis.

Overall, drinking smoothies can be a great way to manage the symptoms of colitis. Smoothies are a convenient and tasty way to get the nutrients your body needs, while also helping to reduce inflammation.

CHAPTER THREE

Smoothie recipes for colitis disease

1. Blueberry Banana Smoothie:

Ingredients:

- ½ cup fresh blueberries

- ½ banana, sliced

- ½ cup plain Greek yogurt

- 1 tablespoon honey

- ½ cup milk

- 1 teaspoon chia seeds

Instructions:

1. Place all ingredients in a blender

2. Blend until smooth

3. Serve and enjoy!

2. Mango Pineapple Smoothie:

Ingredients:

- ½ cup frozen mango

- ½ cup frozen pineapple

- ¼ cup plain Greek yogurt

- 2 tablespoons honey

- ½ cup milk

- 1 teaspoon chia seeds

Instructions:

1. Place all ingredients in a blender

2. Blend until smooth

3. Serve and enjoy!

3. Peanut Butter Banana Smoothie:

Ingredients:

- ½ banana, sliced

- 2 tablespoons peanut butter

- ¼ cup plain Greek yogurt

- 2 tablespoons honey

- ½ cup milk

- 1 teaspoon chia seeds

Instructions:

1. Place all ingredients in a blender

2. Blend until smooth

3. Serve and enjoy!

4. Carrot Orange Smoothie:

Ingredients:

- ½ cup carrots, grated

- ½ cup orange juice

- ¼ cup plain Greek yogurt

- 2 tablespoons honey

- ½ cup milk

- 1 teaspoon chia seeds

Instructions:

1. Place all ingredients in a blender

2. Blend until smooth

3. Serve and enjoy!

5. Avocado Mango Smoothie:

Ingredients:

- ½ cup frozen mango

- ½ avocado, pitted and peeled

- ¼ cup plain Greek yogurt

- 2 tablespoons honey

- ½ cup milk

- 1 teaspoon chia seeds

Instructions:

1. Place all ingredients in a blender

2. Blend until smooth

3. Serve and enjoy!

6. Green Apple Smoothie:

Ingredients:

- ½ green apple, cored and sliced

- ½ cup plain Greek yogurt

- 2 tablespoons honey

- ½ cup milk

- 1 teaspoon chia seeds

Instructions:

1. Place all ingredients in a blender

2. Blend until smooth

3. Serve and enjoy!

7. Spinach Strawberry Smoothie:

Ingredients:

- ½ cup spinach

- ½ cup frozen strawberries

- ¼ cup plain Greek yogurt

- 2 tablespoons honey

- ½ cup milk

- 1 teaspoon chia seeds

Instructions:

1. Place all ingredients in a blender

2. Blend until smooth

3. Serve and enjoy!

8. Kiwi Coconut Smoothie:

Ingredients:

- ½ cup kiwi, peeled and sliced

- ½ cup coconut milk

- ¼ cup plain Greek yogurt

- 2 tablespoons honey

- ½ cup milk

- 1 teaspoon chia seeds

Instructions:

1. Place all ingredients in a blender

2. Blend until smooth

3. Serve and enjoy!

9. Pineapple Banana Smoothie:

Ingredients:

- ½ cup pineapple, chopped

- ½ banana, sliced

- ¼ cup plain Greek yogurt

- 2 tablespoons honey

- ½ cup milk

- 1 teaspoon chia seeds

Instructions:

1. Place all ingredients in a blender

2. Blend until smooth

3. Serve and enjoy!

10. Beet Apple Smoothie:

Ingredients:

- ½ cup beets, cooked and chopped

- ½ green apple, cored and sliced

- ¼ cup plain Greek yogurt

- 2 tablespoons honey

- ½ cup milk

- 1 teaspoon chia seeds

Instructions:

1. Place all ingredients in a blender

2. Blend until smooth

3. Serve and enjoy!

11. Kale Orange Smoothie:

Ingredients:

- ½ cup kale

- ½ cup orange juice

- ¼ cup plain Greek yogurt

- 2 tablespoons honey

- ½ cup milk

- 1 teaspoon chia seeds

Instructions:

1. Place all ingredients in a blender

2. Blend until smooth

3. Serve and enjoy!

12. Papaya Coconut Smoothie:

Ingredients:

- ½ cup papaya, diced

- ½ cup coconut milk

- ¼ cup plain Greek yogurt

- 2 tablespoons honey

- ½ cup milk

- 1 teaspoon chia seeds

Instructions:

1. Place all ingredients in a blender

2. Blend until smooth

3. Serve and enjoy!

13. Peach Almond Smoothie:

Ingredients:

- ½ cup frozen peaches

- 2 tablespoons almond butter

- ¼ cup plain Greek yogurt

- 2 tablespoons honey

- ½ cup milk

- 1 teaspoon chia seeds

Instructions:

1. Place all ingredients in a blender

2. Blend until smooth

3. Serve and enjoy!

14. Carrot Orange Ginger Smoothie:

Ingredients:

- ½ cup carrots, grated

- ½ cup orange juice

- ½ teaspoon ginger, grated

- ¼ cup plain Greek yogurt

- 2 tablespoons honey

- ½ cup milk

- 1 teaspoon chia seeds

Instructions:

1. Place all ingredients in a blender

2. Blend until smooth

3. Serve and enjoy!

15. Apple Cinnamon Smoothie:

Ingredients:

- ½ green apple, cored and sliced

- ½ teaspoon cinnamon

- ¼ cup plain Greek yogurt

- 2 tablespoons honey

- ½ cup milk

- 1 teaspoon chia seeds

Instructions:

1. Place all ingredients in a blender

2. Blend until smooth

3. Serve and enjoy!

16. Banana Oat Smoothie:

Ingredients:

- ½ banana, sliced

- 2 tablespoons oats

- ¼ cup plain Greek yogurt

- 2 tablespoons honey

- ½ cup milk

- 1 teaspoon chia seeds

Instructions:

1. Place all ingredients in a blender

2. Blend until smooth

3. Serve and enjoy!

17. Strawberry Coconut Smoothie:

Ingredients:

- ½ cup frozen strawberries

- ½ cup coconut milk

- ¼ cup plain Greek yogurt

- 2 tablespoons honey

- ½ cup milk

- 1 teaspoon chia seeds

Instructions:

1. Place all ingredients in a blender

2. Blend until smooth

3. Serve and enjoy!

18. Watermelon Mint Smoothie:

Ingredients:

- ½ cup watermelon, diced

- 1 teaspoon mint leaves

- ¼ cup plain Greek yogurt

- 2 tablespoons honey

- ½ cup milk

- 1 teaspoon chia seeds

Instructions:

1. Place all ingredients in a blender

2. Blend until smooth

3. Serve and enjoy!

19. Kale Banana Smoothie:

Ingredients:

- ½ cup kale

- ½ banana, sliced

- ¼ cup plain Greek yogurt

- 2 tablespoons honey

- ½ cup milk

- 1 teaspoon chia seeds

Instructions:

1. Place all ingredients in a blender

2. Blend until smooth

3. Serve and enjoy!

20. Avocado Pineapple Smoothie:

Ingredients:

- ½ avocado, pitted and peeled

- ½ cup frozen pineapple

- ¼ cup plain Greek yogurt

- 2 tablespoons honey

- ½ cup milk

- 1 teaspoon chia seeds

Instructions:

1. Place all ingredients in a blender

2. Blend until smooth

3. Serve and enjoy!

21. Blueberry Banana Colitis Smoothie:

Ingredients:

- 1 banana
- ½ cup frozen blueberries
- 1 cup almond milk
- ¼ cup plain Greek yogurt
- 1 teaspoon chia seeds
- 1 teaspoon honey

Instructions:

1. All ingredients should be put in a blender and blend
2. Pour into a glass and enjoy.

22. Pineapple Mango Colitis Smoothie:

Ingredients:

- ½ cup frozen pineapple
- ½ cup frozen mango

- 1 cup almond milk
- 1 tablespoon honey

Instructions:

1. All ingredients should be put in a blender and blend

2. Pour into a glass and enjoy.

23. Spinach Kale Colitis Smoothie:

Ingredients:

- 1 cup fresh spinach
- 1 cup fresh kale
- ½ banana
- 1 cup almond milk
- 1 teaspoon honey
- 1 teaspoon chia seeds

Instructions:

1. All ingredients should be put in a blender and blend

2. Pour into a glass and enjoy.

24. Green Apple Colitis Smoothie:

Ingredients:

- 1 green apple, cored and chopped
- 1 banana
- 1 cup almond milk
- 1 tablespoon honey

Instructions:

1. All ingredients should be put in a blender and blend

2. Pour into a glass and enjoy.

25. Strawberry Banana Colitis Smoothie:

Ingredients:

- ½ cup frozen strawberries
- 1 banana
- 1 cup almond milk
- 1 tablespoon honey

Instructions:

1. All ingredients should be put in a blender and blend

2. Pour into a glass and enjoy.

26. Avocado Pear Colitis Smoothie:

Ingredients:

- ½ avocado
- 1 pear, cored and chopped
- 1 cup almond milk
- 1 tablespoon honey

Instructions:

1. All ingredients should be put in a blender and blend

2. Pour into a glass and enjoy.

27. Coconut Mango Colitis Smoothie:

Ingredients:

- ½ cup frozen mango
- ½ cup coconut milk

- 1 tablespoon honey

Instructions:

1. All ingredients should be put in a blender and blend

2. Pour into a glass and enjoy.

28. Peach Blueberry Colitis Smoothie:

Ingredients:

- ½ cup frozen peaches

- ½ cup frozen blueberries

- 1 cup almond milk

- 1 teaspoon honey

Instructions:

1. All ingredients should be put in a blender and blend

2. Pour into a glass and enjoy.

29. Apple Cinnamon Colitis Smoothie:

Ingredients:

- 1 green apple, cored and chopped
- 1 cup almond milk
- ½ teaspoon ground cinnamon
- 1 tablespoon honey

Instructions:

1. All ingredients should be put in a blender and blend
2. Pour into a glass and enjoy.

30. Lemon Ginger Colitis Smoothie:

Ingredients:

- 1 lemon, juiced
- ½ inch fresh ginger, peeled and grated nicely
- 1 cup almond milk
- 1 teaspoon honey

Instructions:

1. All ingredients should be put in a blender and blend

2. Pour into a glass and enjoy.

31. Orange Carrot Colitis Smoothie:

Ingredients:

- 1 orange, peeled and chopped
- ½ cup carrots, chopped
- 1 cup almond milk
- 1 tablespoon honey

Instructions:

1. All ingredients should be put in a blender and blend

2. Pour into a glass and enjoy.

32. Kale Banana Colitis Smoothie:

Ingredients:

- 1 cup fresh kale
- 1 banana
- 1 cup almond milk

- 1 teaspoon honey

Instructions:

1. All ingredients should be put in a blender and blend

2. Pour into a glass and enjoy.

33. Cucumber Melon Colitis Smoothie:

Ingredients:

- ½ cup cucumber, chopped
- ½ cup frozen melon
- 1 cup almond milk
- 1 tablespoon honey

Instructions:

1. All ingredients should be put in a blender and blend

2. Pour into a glass and enjoy.

34. Pineapple Coconut Colitis Smoothie:

Ingredients:

- ½ cup frozen pineapple
- ½ cup coconut milk
- 1 teaspoon honey

Instructions:

1. All ingredients should be put in a blender and blend
2. Pour into a glass and enjoy.

35. Acai Berry Colitis Smoothie:

Ingredients:

- ½ cup frozen acai berries
- 1 banana
- 1 cup almond milk
- 1 tablespoon honey

Instructions:

1. All ingredients should be put in a blender and blend

2. Pour into a glass and enjoy.

36. Mango Coconut Colitis Smoothie:

Ingredients:

- ½ cup frozen mango
- ½ cup coconut milk
- 1 tablespoon honey

Instructions:

1. All ingredients should be put in a blender and blend

2. Pour into a glass and enjoy.

37. Banana Almond Butter Colitis Smoothie:

Ingredients:

- 1 banana
- 1 cup almond milk
- 1 tablespoon almond butter
- 1 teaspoon honey

Instructions:

1. All ingredients should be put in a blender and blend

2. Pour into a glass and enjoy.

38. Carrot Orange Colitis Smoothie:

Ingredients:

- ½ cup carrots, chopped
- 1 orange, peeled and chopped
- 1 cup almond milk
- 1 tablespoon honey

Instructions:

1. All ingredients should be put in a blender and blend

2. Pour into a glass and enjoy.

39. Peach Coconut Colitis Smoothie:

Ingredients:

- ½ cup frozen peaches
- ½ cup coconut milk
- 1 teaspoon honey

Instructions:

1. All ingredients should be put in a blender and blend

2. Pour into a glass and enjoy.

40. Strawberry Coconut Colitis Smoothie:

Ingredients:

- ½ cup frozen strawberries
- ½ cup coconut milk
- 1 tablespoon honey

Instructions:

1. All ingredients should be put in a blender and blend

2. Pour into a glass and enjoy.

41. Green Colitis Smoothie:

Ingredients:

- 1 cup of almond milk
- 1 banana
- 1/2 cup spinach

- 1/2 cup kale

- 1 tablespoon chia seed

- 1 teaspoon honey

Instructions:

1. All ingredients should be put in a blender and blend

2. Pour into a glass and enjoy!

42. Mango Turmeric Smoothie:

Ingredients:

- 1 cup of almond milk

- 1 cup of mango

- 1 teaspoon turmeric

- 1 tablespoon of hemp seeds

- 1 tablespoon of chia seeds

- 1/4 teaspoon of cinnamon

Instructions:

1. All ingredients should be put in a blender and blend

2. Pour into a glass and enjoy!

43. Blueberry Ginger Smoothie:

Ingredients:

- 1 cup of almond milk

- 1 cup of blueberries

- 1 tablespoon of ginger

- 1 teaspoon of honey

- 1 tablespoon of chia seeds

- 1/2 teaspoon of cinnamon

Instructions:

1. All ingredients should be put in a blender and blend

2. Pour into a glass and enjoy!

44. Coconut Berry Smoothie:

Ingredients:

- 1 cup of coconut milk

- 1/2 cup of raspberries

- 1/2 cup of blueberries

- 1 teaspoon of honey

- 1 tablespoon of chia seeds

- 1 teaspoon of cinnamon

Instructions:

1. All ingredients should be put in a blender and blend

2. Pour into a glass and enjoy!

45. Avocado Spinach Smoothie:

Ingredients:

- 1 cup of almond milk

- 1/2 avocado

- 1/2 cup spinach

- 1 teaspoon of honey

- 1 tablespoon of chia seeds

- 1/4 teaspoon of cinnamon

Instructions:

1. All ingredients should be put in a blender and blend

2. Pour into a glass and enjoy!

46. Broccoli Beet Smoothie:

Ingredients:

- 1 cup of almond milk
- 1/2 cup of broccoli
- 1/2 cup of beets
- 1 teaspoon of honey
- 1 tablespoon of chia seeds
- 1/4 teaspoon of cinnamon

Instructions:

1. All ingredients should be put in a blender and blend

2. Pour into a glass and enjoy!

47. Carrot Apple Smoothie:

Ingredients:

- 1 cup of almond milk
- 1/2 cup of carrots
- 1/2 cup of apples

- 1 teaspoon of honey

- 1 tablespoon of chia seeds

- 1/4 teaspoon of cinnamon

Instructions:

1. All ingredients should be put in a blender and blend

2. Pour into a glass and enjoy!

48. Kale Pineapple Smoothie:

Ingredients:

- 1 cup of almond milk

- 1/2 cup of kale

- 1/2 cup of pineapple

- 1 teaspoon of honey

- 1 tablespoon of chia seeds

- 1/4 teaspoon of cinnamon

Instructions:

1. All ingredients should be put in a blender and blend

2. Pour into a glass and enjoy!

49. Banana Oat Smoothie:

Ingredients:

- 1 cup of almond milk

- 1 banana

- 1/4 cup of oats

- 1 teaspoon of honey

- 1 tablespoon of chia seeds

- 1/4 teaspoon of cinnamon

Instructions:

1. All ingredients should be put in a blender and blend

2. Pour into a glass and enjoy!

50. Sweet Potato Cucumber Smoothie:

Ingredients:

- 1 cup of almond milk

- 1/2 cup of sweet potatoes

- 1/2 cup of cucumbers
- 1 teaspoon of honey
- 1 tablespoon of chia seeds
- 1/4 teaspoon of cinnamon

Instructions:

1. All ingredients should be put in a blender and blend
2. Pour into a glass and enjoy!

51. Carrot Orange Smoothie:

Ingredients:

- 1 cup of almond milk
- 1/2 cup of carrots
- 1/2 cup of oranges
- 1 teaspoon of honey
- 1 tablespoon of chia seeds
- 1/4 teaspoon of cinnamon

Instructions:

1. All ingredients should be put in a blender and blend

2. Pour into a glass and enjoy!

52. Kale Coconut Smoothie:

Ingredients:

- 1 cup of coconut milk
- 1/2 cup of kale
- 1 tablespoon of coconut oil
- 1 teaspoon of honey
- 1 tablespoon of chia seeds
- 1/4 teaspoon of cinnamon

Instructions:

1. All ingredients should be put in a blender and blend

2. Pour into a glass and enjoy!

53. Spinach Mango Smoothie:

Ingredients:

- 1 cup of almond milk

- 1/2 cup of spinach
- 1/2 cup of mango
- 1 teaspoon of honey
- 1 tablespoon of chia seeds
- 1/4 teaspoon of cinnamon

Instructions:

1. All ingredients should be put in a blender and blend
2. Pour into a glass and enjoy!

54. Beet Ginger Smoothie:

Ingredients:

- 1 cup of almond milk
- 1/2 cup of beets
- 1 tablespoon of ginger
- 1 teaspoon of honey
- 1 tablespoon of chia seeds
- 1/4 teaspoon of cinnamon

Instructions:

1. All ingredients should be put in a blender and blend

2. Pour into a glass and enjoy!

55. Apple Banana Smoothie:

Ingredients:

- 1 cup of almond milk
- 1/2 cup of apples
- 1 banana
- 1 teaspoon of honey
- 1 tablespoon of chia seeds
- 1/4 teaspoon of cinnamon

Instructions:

1. All ingredients should be put in a blender and blend

2. Pour into a glass and enjoy!

56. Cucumber Pineapple Smoothie:

Ingredients:

- 1 cup of almond milk

- 1/2 cup of cucumbers
- 1/2 cup of pineapple
- 1 teaspoon of honey
- 1 tablespoon of chia seeds
- 1/4 teaspoon of cinnamon

Instructions:

1. All ingredients should be put in a blender and blend
2. Pour into a glass and enjoy!

57. Avocado Turmeric Smoothie:

Ingredients:

- 1 cup of almond milk
- 1/2 avocado
- 1 teaspoon of turmeric
- 1 teaspoon of honey
- 1 tablespoon of chia seeds
- 1/4 teaspoon of cinnamon

Instructions:

1. All ingredients should be put in a blender and blend

2. Pour into a glass and enjoy!

58. Strawberry Hemp Smoothie:

Ingredients:

- 1 cup of almond milk
- 1 cup of strawberries
- 1 tablespoon of hemp seeds
- 1 teaspoon of honey
- 1 tablespoon of chia seeds
- 1/4 teaspoon of cinnamon

Instructions:

1. All ingredients should be put in a blender and blend

2. Pour into a glass and enjoy!

59. Broccoli Coconut Smoothie:

Ingredients:

- 1 cup of coconut milk

- 1/2 cup of broccoli
- 1 tablespoon of coconut oil
- 1 teaspoon of honey
- 1 tablespoon of chia seeds
- 1/4 teaspoon of cinnamon

Instructions:

1. All ingredients should be put in a blender and blend
2. Pour into a glass and enjoy!

60. Banana Chia Smoothie:

Ingredients:

- 1 cup of almond milk
- 1 banana
- 1 tablespoon of chia seeds
- 1 teaspoon of honey
- 1/4 teaspoon of cinnamon

Instructions:

1. All ingredients should be put in a blender and blend

2. Pour into a glass and enjoy!

61. Tropical Colitis Smoothie -

Ingredients:

1 banana,

2 cups pineapple,

1 cup coconut milk,

1 cup spinach,

1 tablespoon honey

Instructions:

1. All ingredients should be put in a blender and blend

2. Pour into a glass and enjoy!

62. Blueberry-Mango Colitis Smoothie -

Ingredients:

1 cup frozen blueberries,

1 cup frozen mango,

2 cups almond milk,

1 tablespoon chia seeds,

1 tablespoon ground flaxseed

Instructions:

1. All ingredients should be put in a blender and blend

2. Pour into a glass and enjoy!

63. Green Colitis Smoothie -

Ingredients:

1 cup spinach,

1 cup kale,

1 cup apple juice,

1 tablespoon almond butter,

1 tablespoon ground flaxseed

Instructions:

1. All ingredients should be put in a blender and blend

2. Pour into a glass and enjoy!

64. Coconut Colitis Smoothie -
Ingredients:

2 cups coconut milk,

2 tablespoons shredded coconut,

1 banana,

1 tablespoon chia seeds,

1 tablespoon honey

Instructions:

2. All ingredients should be put in a blender and blend

2. Pour into a glass and enjoy!

65. Strawberry Colitis Smoothie -
Ingredients:

2 cups strawberries,

1 cup apple juice,

1 cup almond milk,

1 tablespoon chia seeds,

1 tablespoon ground flaxseed

Instructions:

1. All ingredients should be put in a blender and blend

2. Pour into a glass and enjoy!

66. Citrus Colitis Smoothie -
Ingredients:

1 cup orange juice,

1 cup pineapple juice,

1 banana,

1 tablespoon chia seeds,

1 tablespoon honey

Instructions:

1. All ingredients should be put in a blender and blend

2. Pour into a glass and enjoy!

67. Pineapple Colitis Smoothie -
Ingredients:

1 cup pineapple,

1 banana,

1 cup almond milk,

1 tablespoon ground flaxseed,

1 tablespoon honey

Instructions:

1. All ingredients should be put in a blender and blend

2. Pour into a glass and enjoy!

68. Avocado Colitis Smoothie -
Ingredients:

1 avocado,

1 banana,

1 cup coconut milk,

1 tablespoon chia seeds,

1 tablespoon honey

Instructions:

- All ingredients should be put in a blender and blend

2. Pour into a glass and enjoy!

69. Acai Colitis Smoothie -

Ingredients:

1 cup frozen acai berries,

1 banana,

1 cup almond milk,

1 tablespoon chia seeds,

1 tablespoon honey

Instructions:

1. All ingredients should be put in a blender and blend

2. Pour into a glass and enjoy!

70. Mango Colitis Smoothie -

Ingredients:

1 cup frozen mango,

1 banana,

1 cup coconut milk,

1 tablespoon ground flaxseed,

1 tablespoon honey

Instructions:

1. All ingredients should be put in a blender and blend

2. Pour into a glass and enjoy!

71. Papaya Colitis Smoothie -

Ingredients:

1 cup diced papaya,

1 banana,

1 cup almond milk,

1 tablespoon chia seeds,

1 tablespoon honey

Instructions:

1. All ingredients should be put in a blender and blend

2. Pour into a glass and enjoy!

72. Peach Colitis Smoothie -

Ingredients:

1 cup frozen peaches,

1 banana,

1 cup almond milk,

1 tablespoon ground flaxseed,

1 tablespoon honey

Instructions:

1. All ingredients should be put in a blender and blend

2. Pour into a glass and enjoy!

73. Watermelon Colitis Smoothie -
Ingredients:

2 cups diced watermelon,

1 banana,

1 cup coconut milk,

1 tablespoon chia seeds,

1 tablespoon honey

Instructions:

1. All ingredients should be put in a blender and blend

2. Pour into a glass and enjoy!

74. Raspberry Colitis Smoothie -
Ingredients:

1 cup frozen raspberries,

1 banana,

1 cup almond milk,

1 tablespoon ground flaxseed,

1 tablespoon honey

Instructions:

1. All ingredients should be put in a blender and blend

2. Pour into a glass and enjoy!

75. Carrot Colitis Smoothie -
Ingredients:

2 carrots,

1 banana,

1 cup almond milk,

1 tablespoon chia seeds,

1 tablespoon honey

Instructions:

1. All ingredients should be put in a blender and blend

2. Pour into a glass and enjoy!

76. Kale Colitis Smoothie -
Ingredients:

2 cups kale,

1 banana,

1 cup coconut milk,

1 tablespoon ground flaxseed,

1 tablespoon honey

Instructions:

1. All ingredients should be put in a blender and blend

2. Pour into a glass and enjoy!

77. Cucumber Colitis Smoothie -
Ingredients:

2 cups diced cucumber,

1 banana,

1 cup almond milk,

1 tablespoon chia seeds,

1 tablespoon honey

Instructions:

1. All ingredients should be put in a blender and blend

2. Pour into a glass and enjoy!

78. Beet Colitis Smoothie -
Ingredients:

2 beets,

1 banana,

1 cup almond milk,

1 tablespoon ground flaxseed,

1 tablespoon honey

Instructions:

1. All ingredients should be put in a blender and blend

- Pour into a glass and enjoy!

79. Grape Colitis Smoothie -

Ingredients:

1 cup grapes,

1 banana,

1 cup coconut milk,

1 tablespoon chia seeds,

1 tablespoon honey

Instructions:

1. All ingredients should be put in a blender and blend

2. Pour into a glass and enjoy!

80. Banana-Spinach Colitis Smoothie -

Ingredients:

2 bananas,

2 cups spinach,

1 cup almond milk,

1 tablespoon ground flaxseed,

1 tablespoon honey

Instructions:

1. All ingredients should be put in a blender and blend

2. Pour into a glass and enjoy!

Conclusion

By incorporating smoothies that are rich in vitamins, minerals, and anti-inflammatory ingredients into your daily diet, you can help reverse the effects of colitis and improve your overall digestive health.

The key is to maintain a balanced and nutritious diet that includes a variety of healthy ingredients. With the help of smoothies, you can get the essential nutrients your body needs to heal and protect itself from the damaging effects of colitis.

With this newfound knowledge, you can take control of your digestive health and make a positive difference in your life. So, start making healthy smoothies today and take control of your digestive health!

Printed in Great Britain
by Amazon